Illustrated Bird Poetry

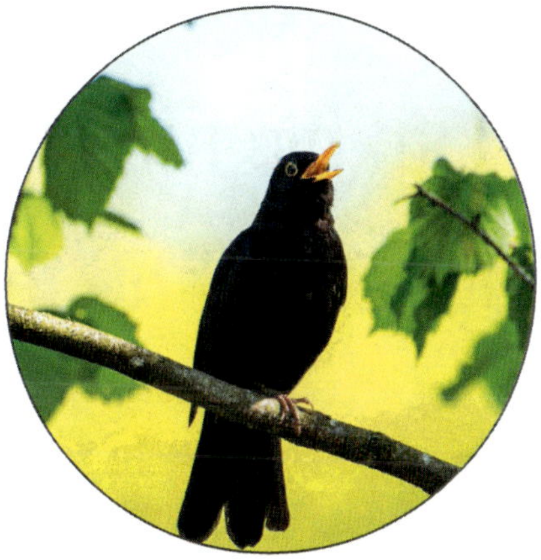

This book of extracts from much-loved classic poems belongs to:

____

The Eagle

He clasps the crag with crooked hands;
Close to the sun in lonely lands,
Ring'd with the azure world, he stands.

The wrinkled sea beneath him crawls;
He watches from his mountain walls,
And like a thunderbolt he falls.

Alfred, Lord Tennyson

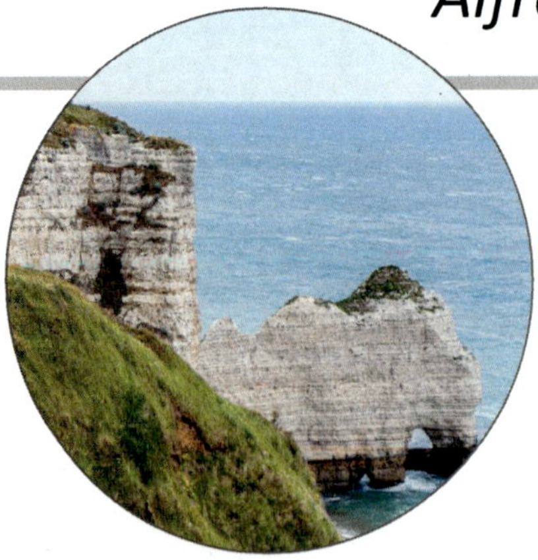

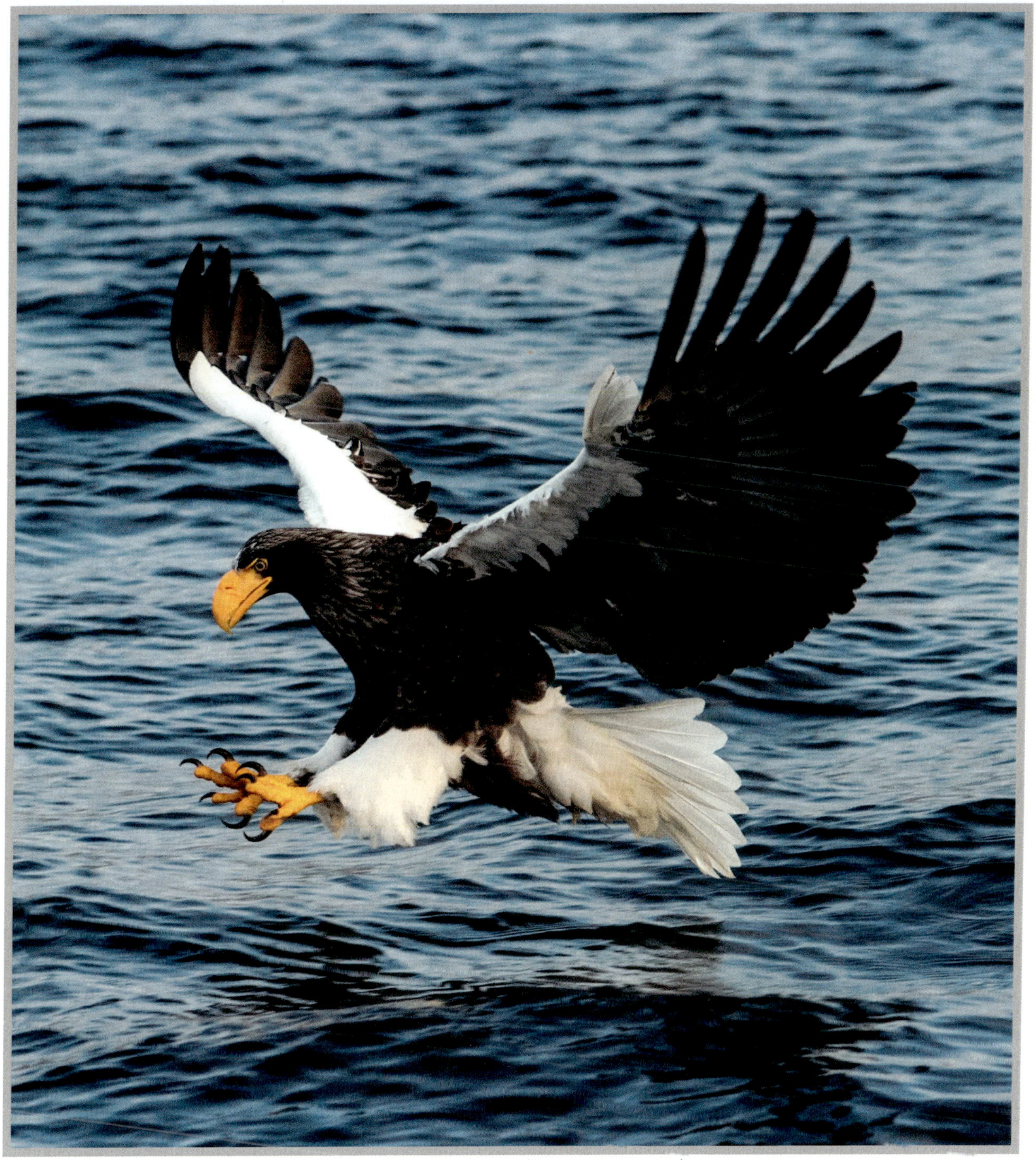

To the Cuckoo

O blithe new-comer! I have heard,
I hear thee and rejoice,
O cuckoo! shall I call thee Bird,
Or but a wandering Voice?

Thrice welcome, darling of the Spring!
Even yet thou art to me
No bird, but an invisible thing,
A voice, a mystery.

William Wordsworth

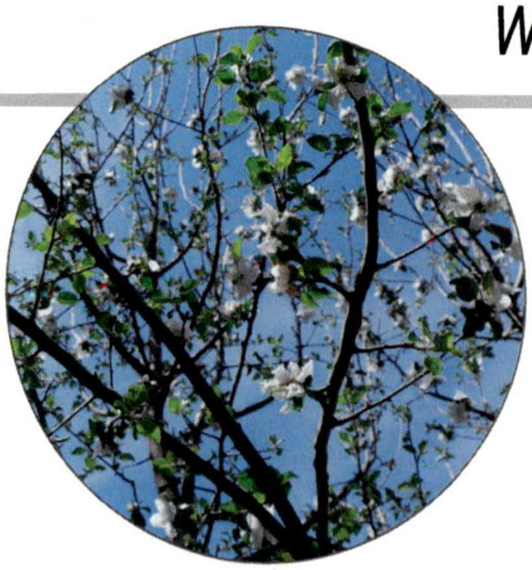

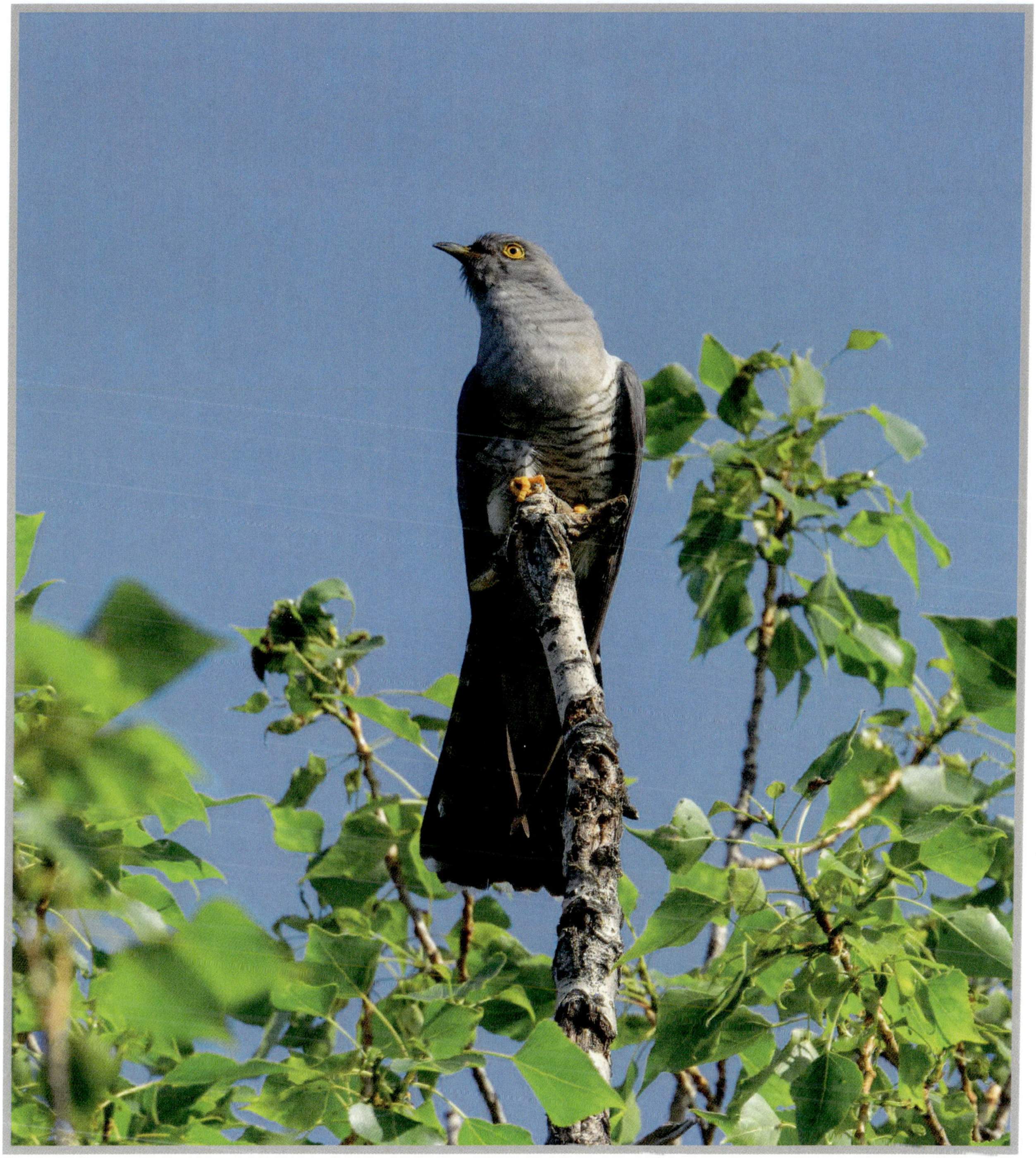

Little Trotty Wagtail

Little Trotty Wagtail
he went in the rain,
And tittering, tottering sideways
he ne'er got straight again,
He stooped to get a worm,
and looked up to get a fly,
And then he flew away
ere his feathers they were dry.

John Clare

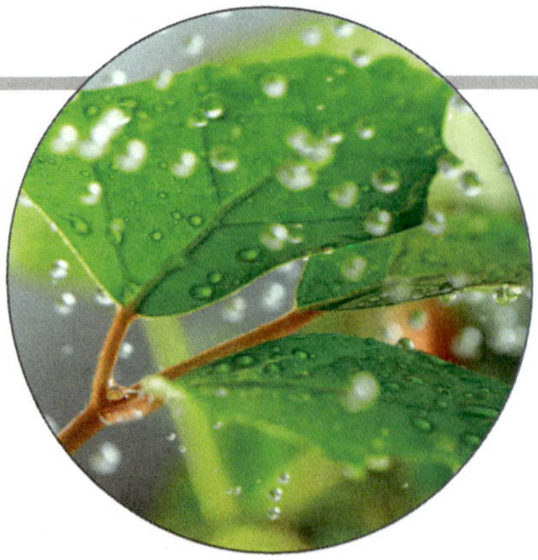

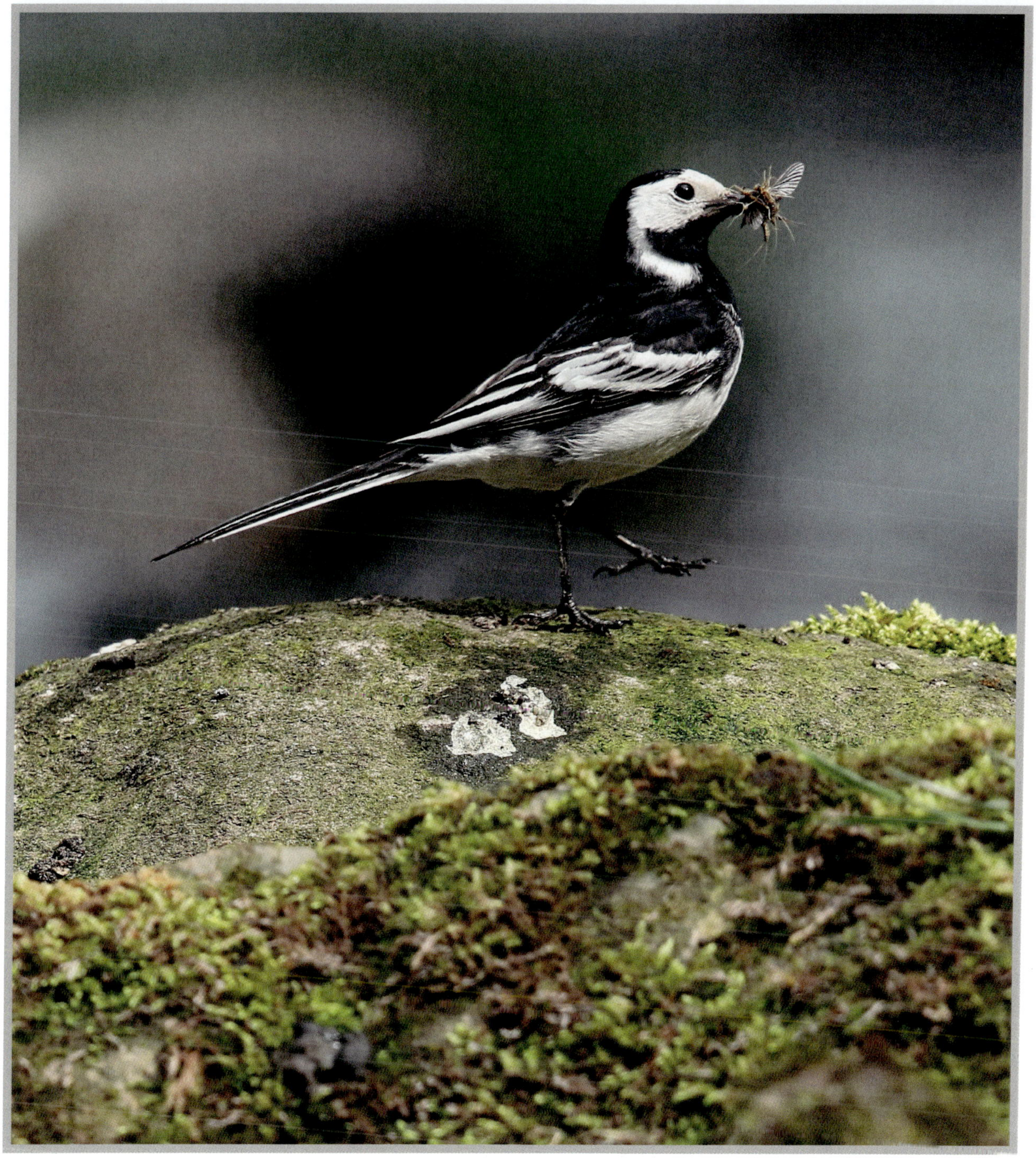

To a Skylark

Hail to thee, blithe Spirit!
Bird thou never wert,
That from Heaven, or near it,
Pourest thy full heart
In profuse strains of unpremeditated art.

Percy Bysshe Shelley

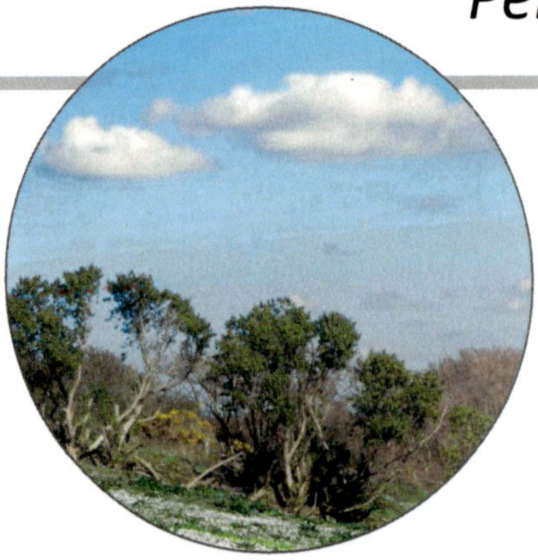

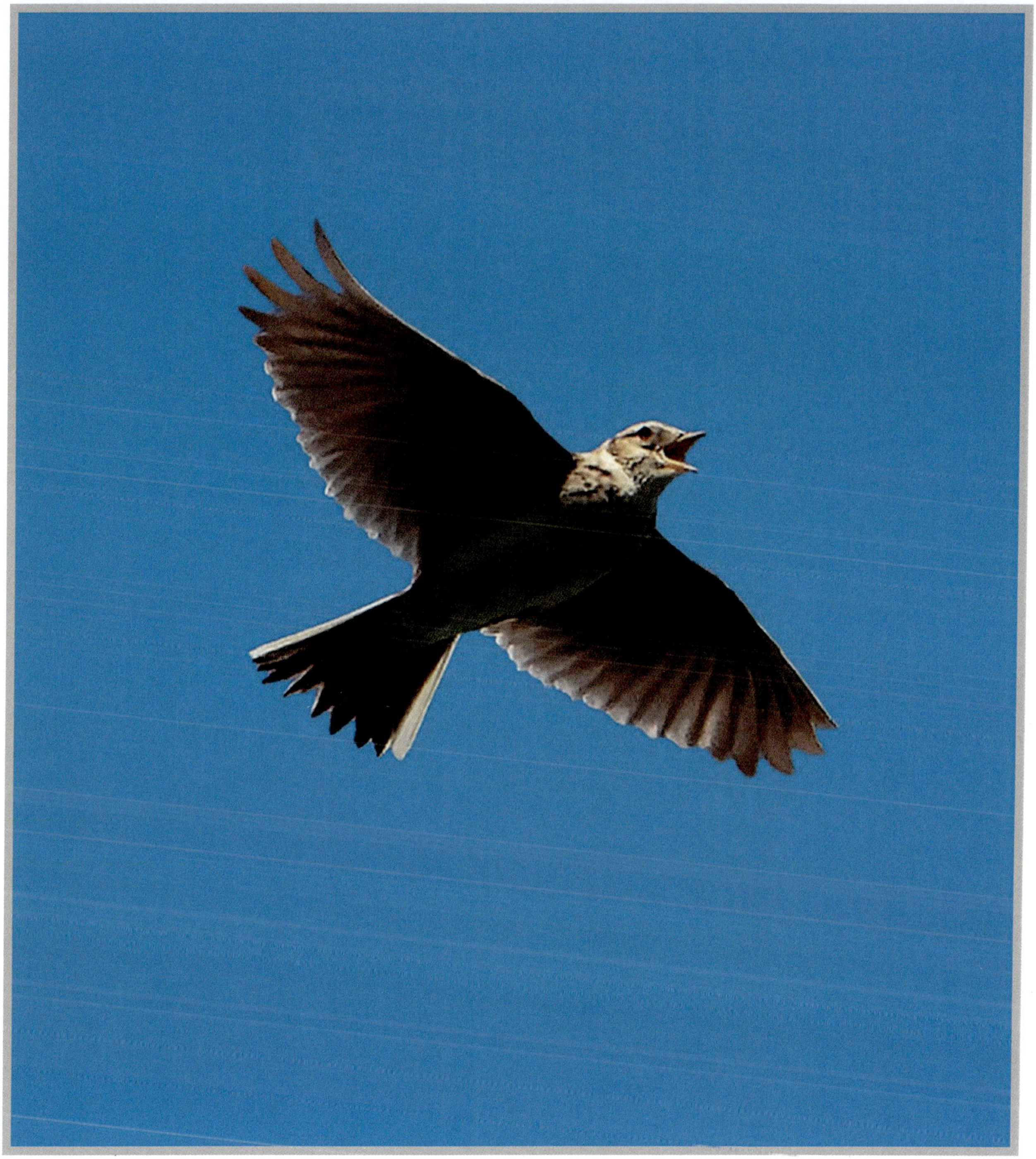

To the Owl

I love to hear thy hooting cry,
At midnight's solemn hour,
On gusty breezes sweeping by,
And feel its utmost power:
From Nature's depths it seems to come,
When other oracles are dumb
And eloquent its sound,
Asserting Night's majestic sway,
And bearing Fancy far away
To solitudes profound.

Bernard Barton

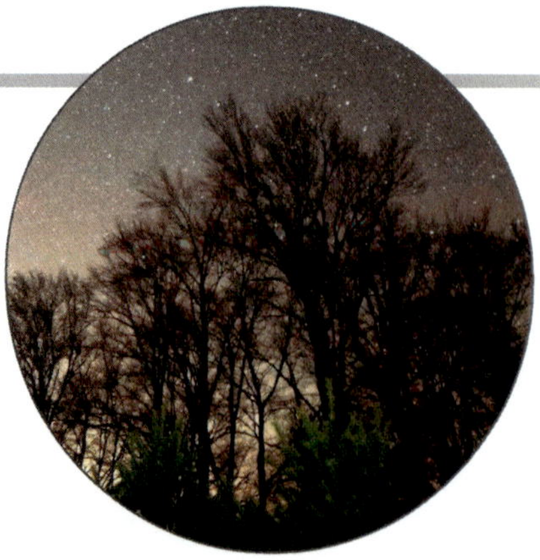

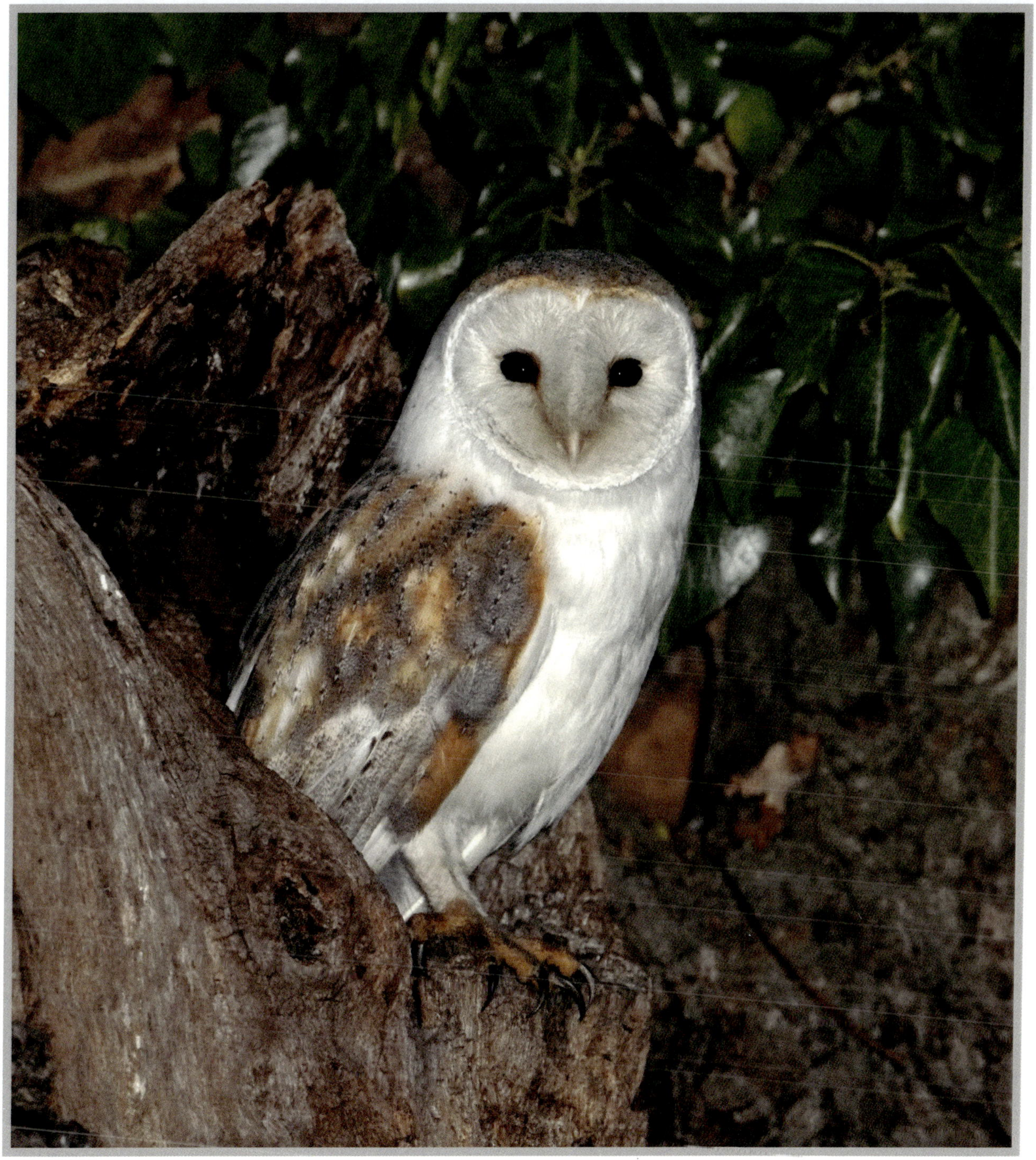

A Bird, came down the Walk

A Bird, came down the Walk -
He did not know I saw -
He bit an Angle Worm in halves
And ate the fellow, raw,

And then, he drank a Dew
From a convenient Grass -
And then hopped sidewise to the Wall
To let a Beetle pass.

Emily Dickinson

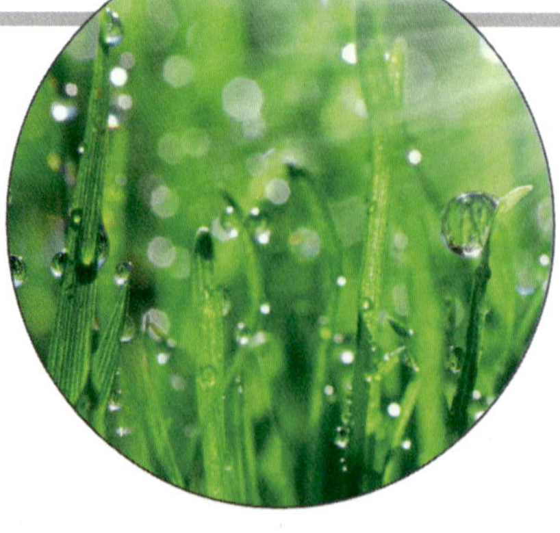

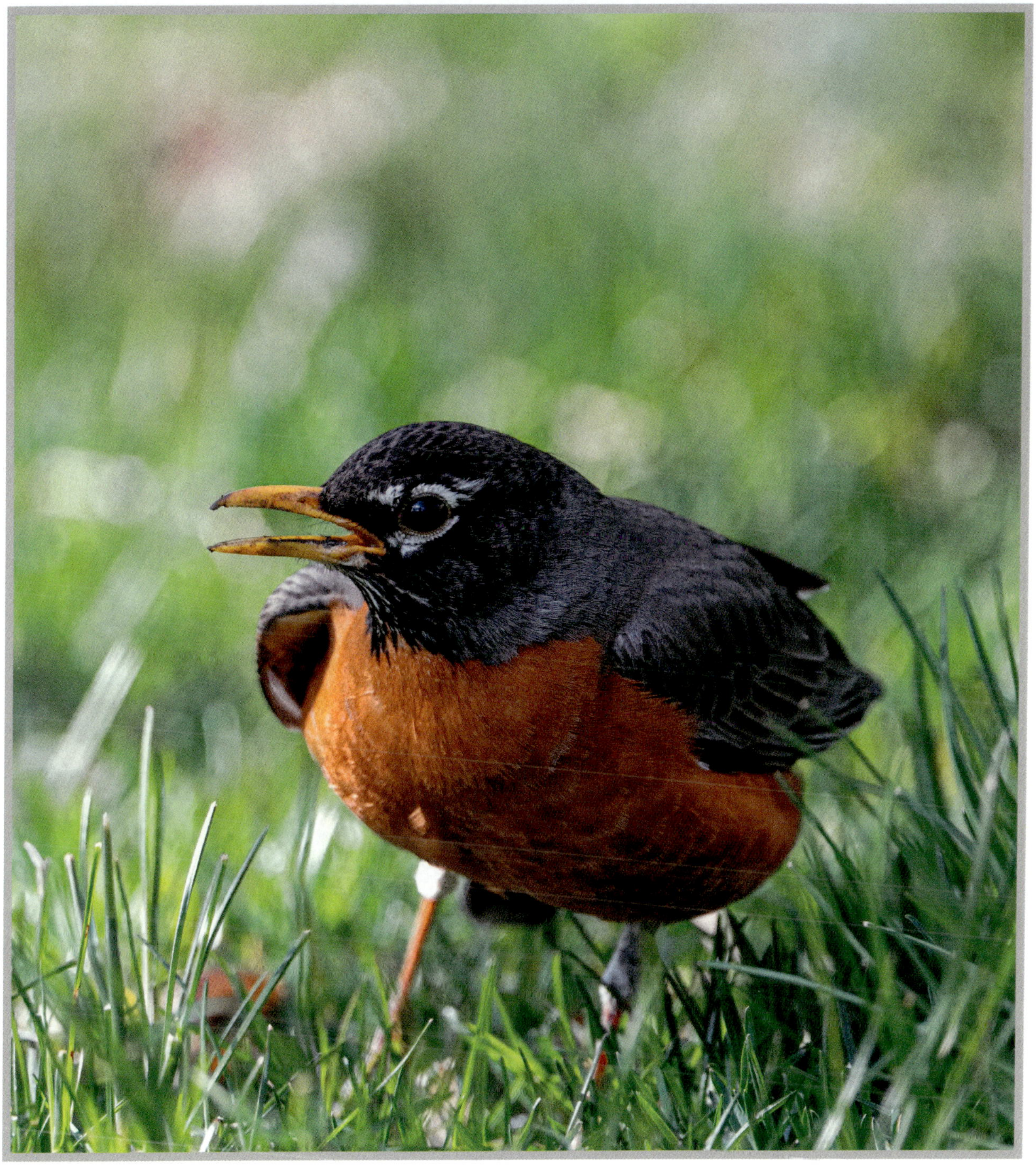

Swallows Travel To and Fro

Swallows travel to and fro,
And the great winds come and go,
And the steady breezes blow,
Bearing perfume, bearing love.
Breezes hasten, swallows fly,
Towered clouds forever ply,
And at noonday, you and I
See the same sunshine above.

Robert Louis Stevenson

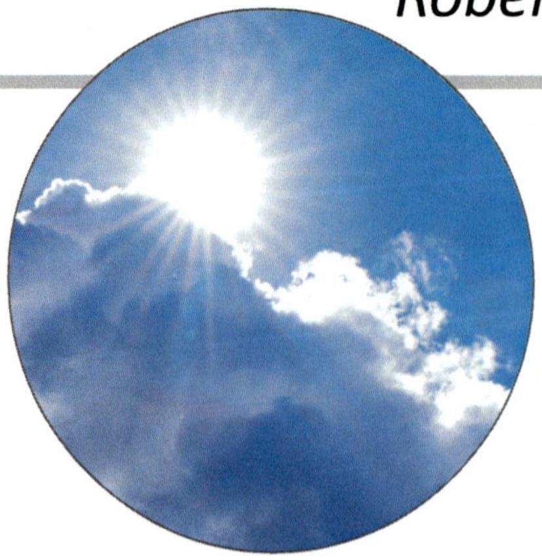

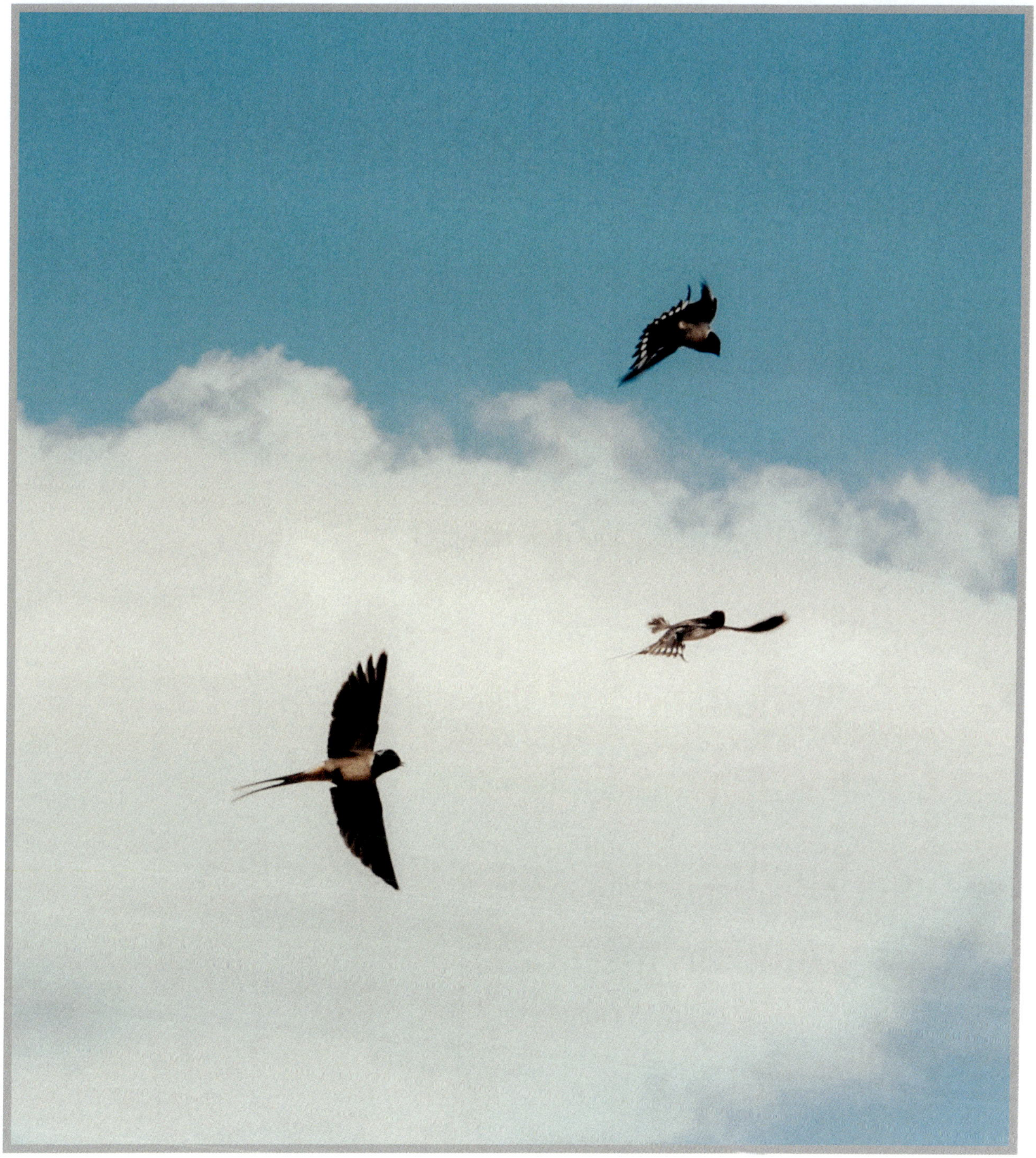

The Wild Geese

Something told the wild geese
It was time to go.
Though the fields lay golden
Something whispered,—'Snow.'

Something told the wild geese
It was time to fly,—
Summer sun was on their wings,
Winter in their cry.

Rachel Field

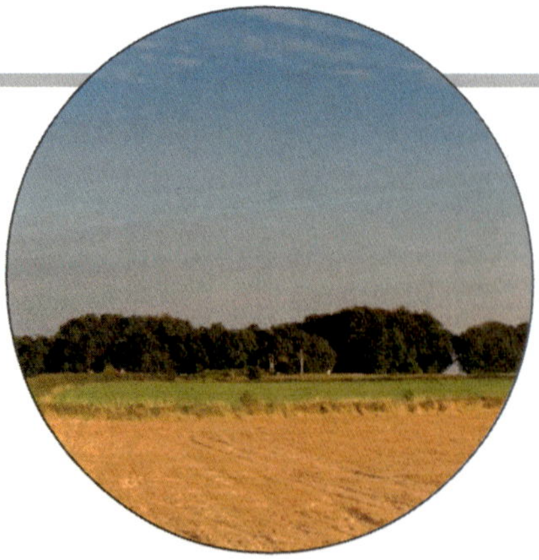

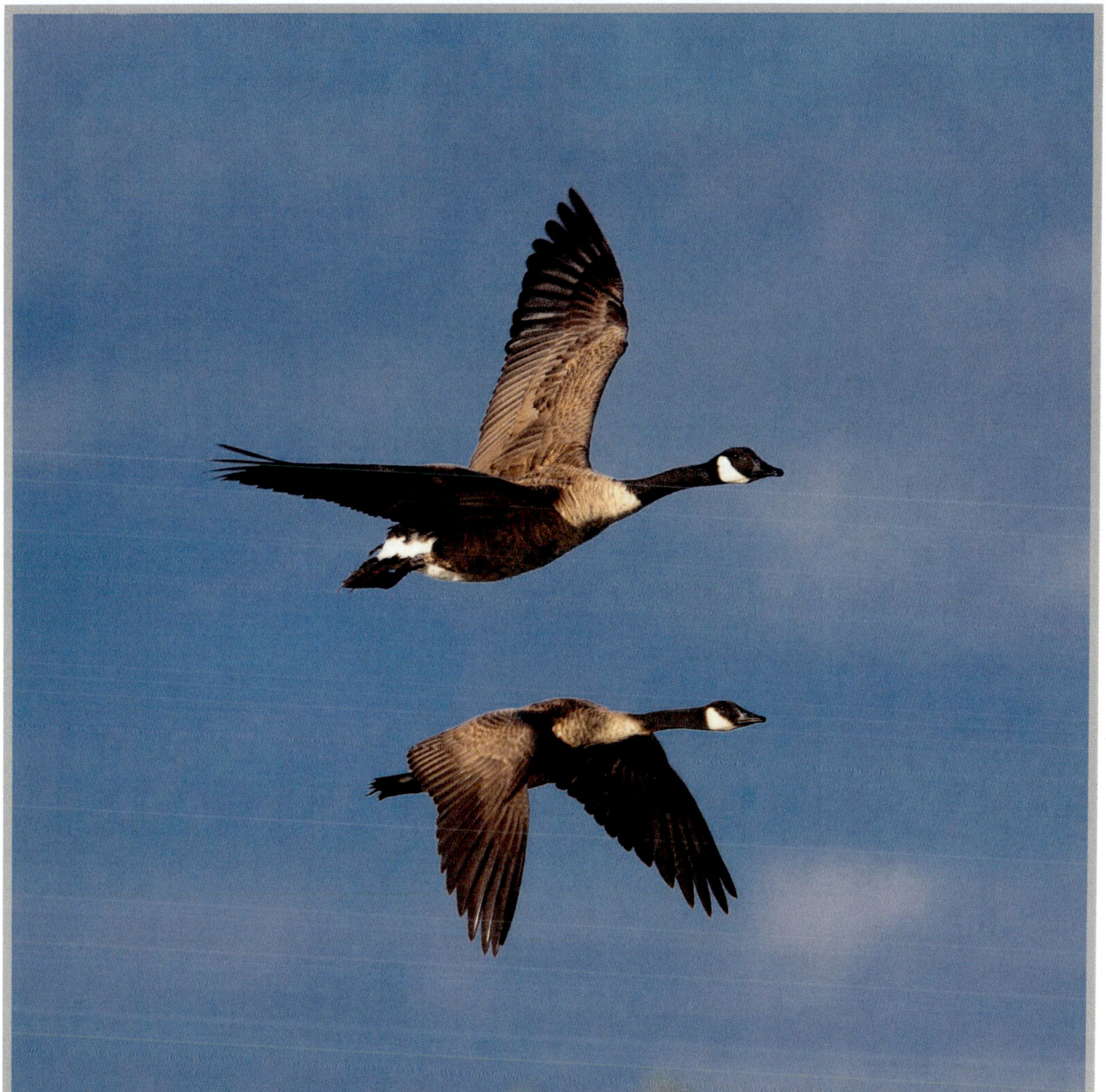

The Swan

Under a wall of bronze,
Where beeches dip and trail
Their branches in the water;
With red-tipped head and wings—
A beaked ship under sail—
There glides a single swan.

John Gould Fletcher

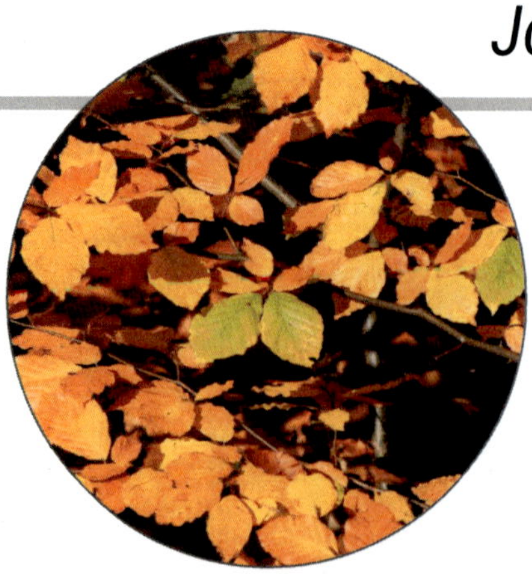

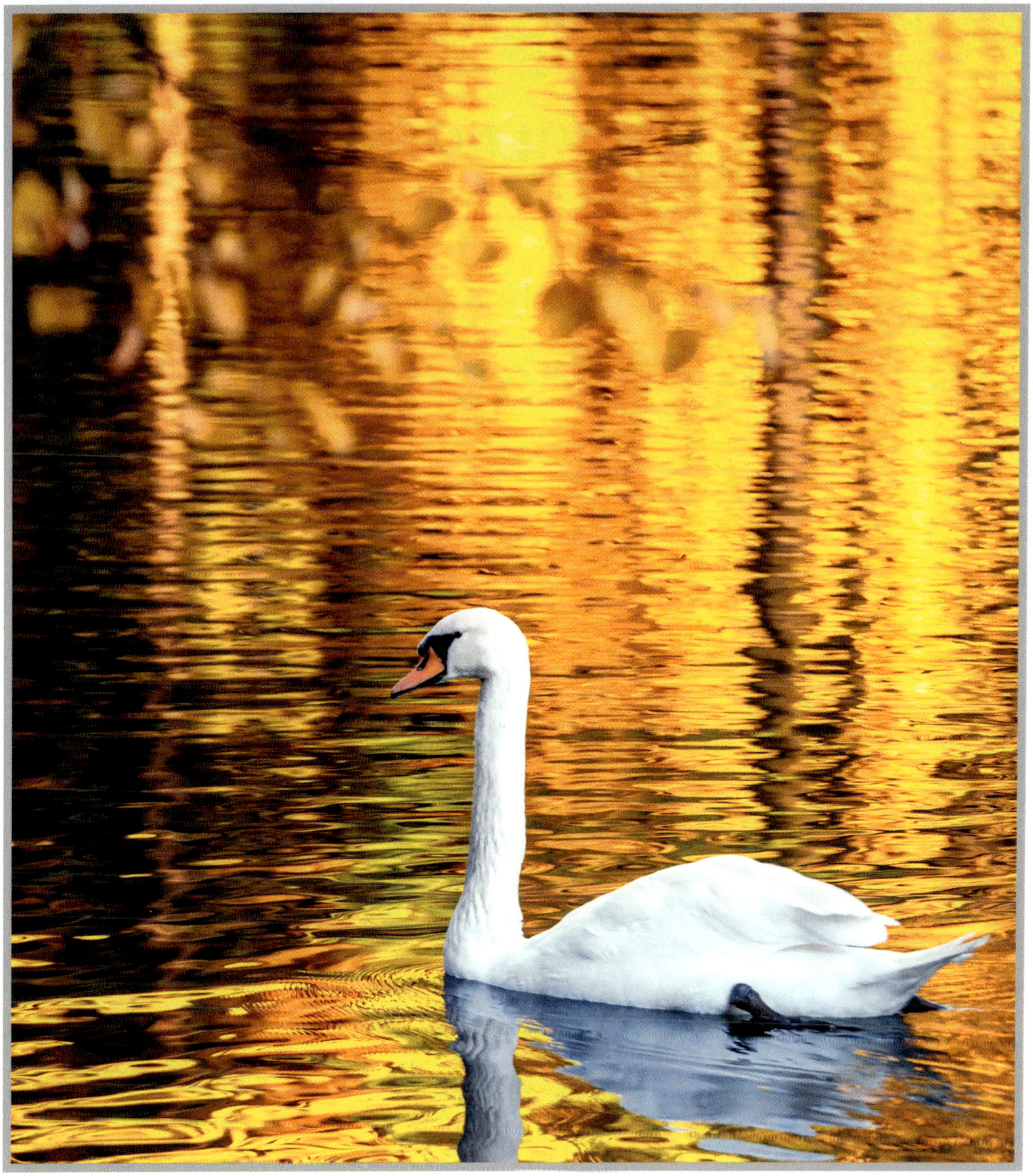

Redbreast

Redbreast, early in the morning
Dank and cold and cloudy grey,
Wildly tender is thy music,
Chasing angry thought away.

Emily Brontë

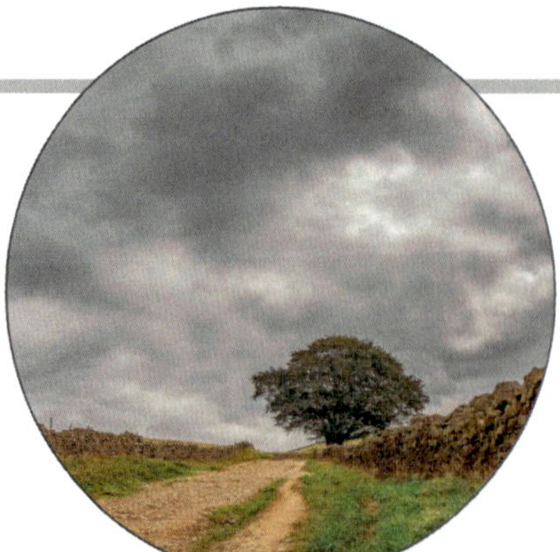

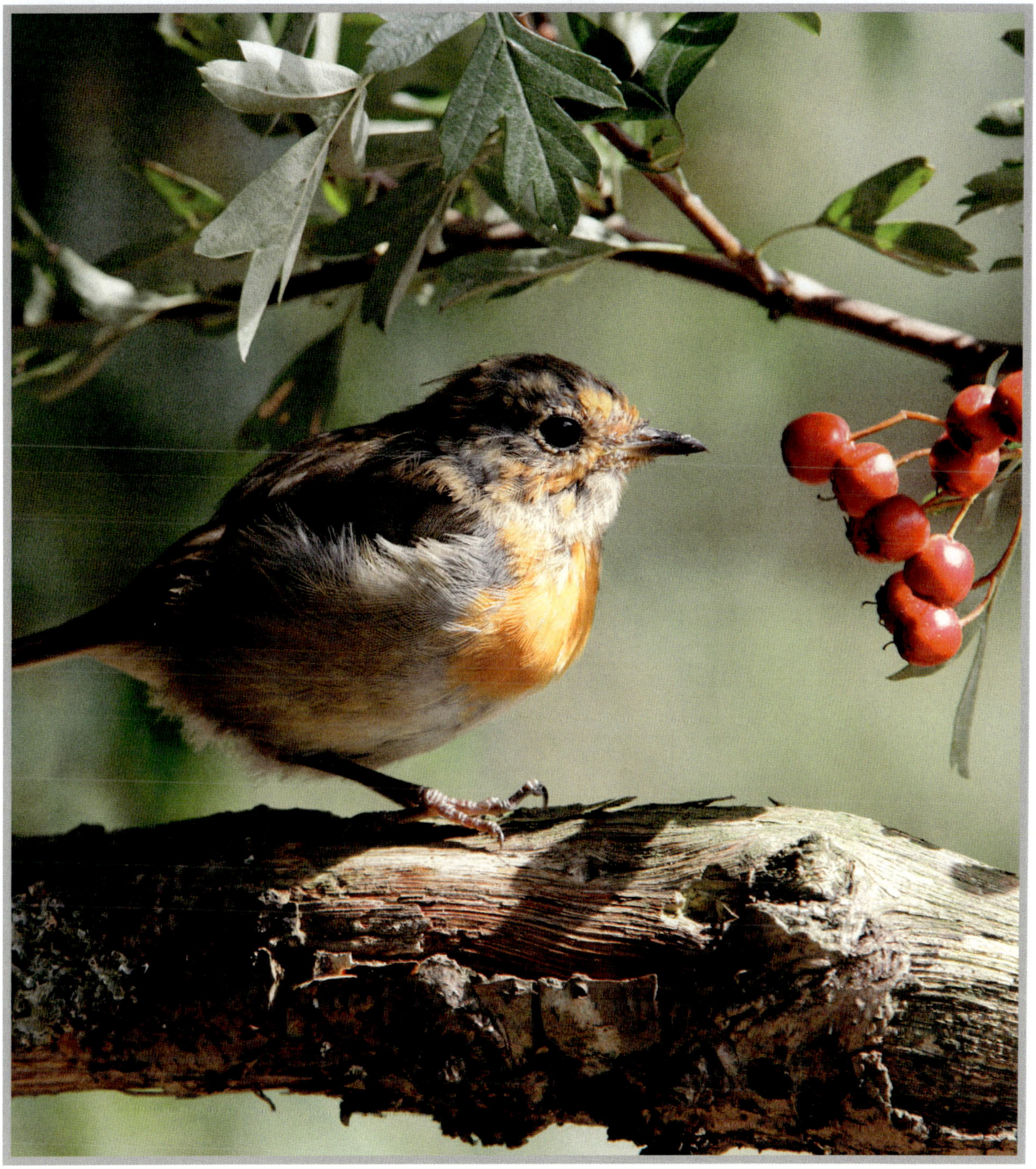

Ducks' Ditty

All along the backwater,
Through the rushes tall,
Ducks are a-dabbling,
Up tails all!

Ducks' tails, drakes' tails,
Yellow feet a-quiver,
Yellow bills all out of sight
Busy in the river!

From
The Wind in the Willows

Kenneth Grahame

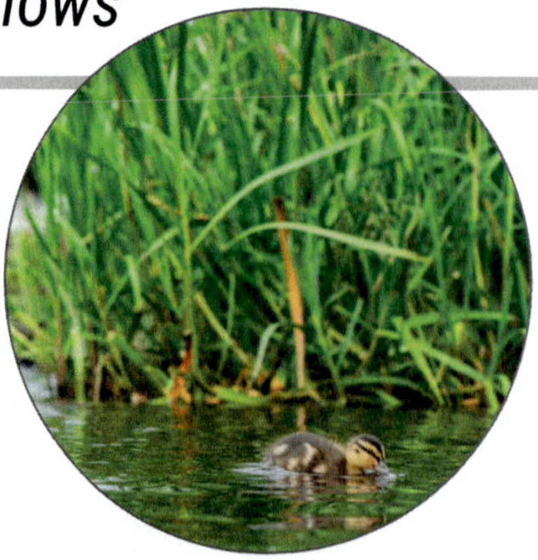

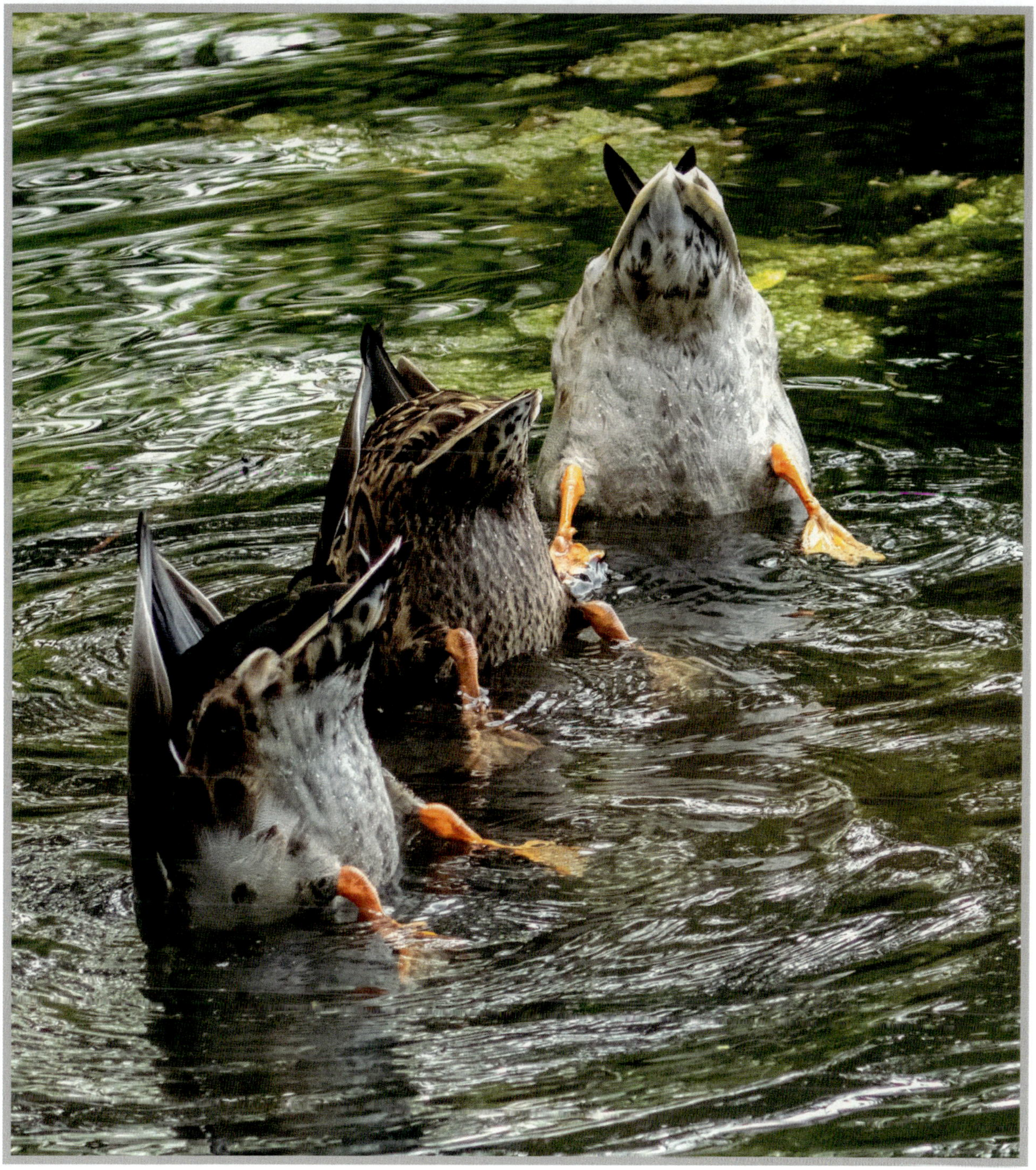

The Cormorant

Now the seagull spreads his wing,
And the puffin seeks the shore,
Home flies every living thing,
Yo, ho! the breakers roar!
Only the cormorant, dark and sly,
Watches the waves with a sea-green eye.

Emily Lawless

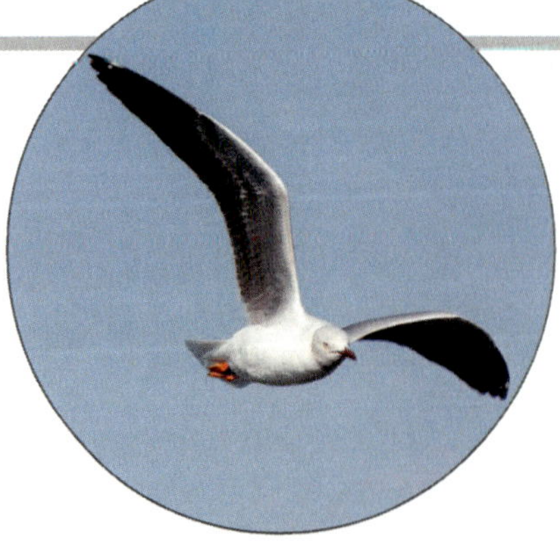

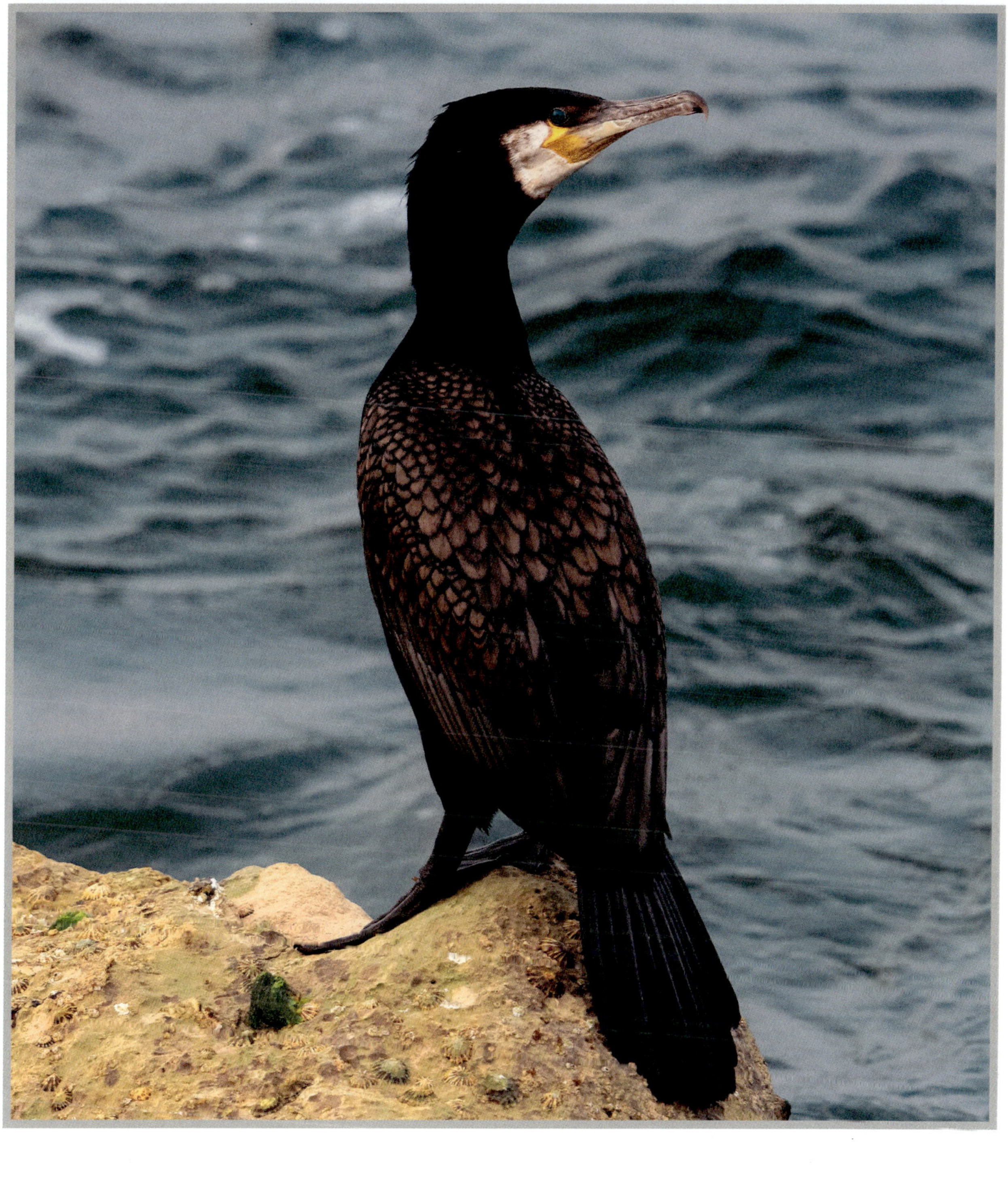

The Return of the Goldfinches

We are much honoured by your choice,
O golden birds of silver voice,
That in our garden you should find
A pleasure to your mind—

First you were spied a flighting pair
Flashing and fluting here and there,
Until in stealth the nest was made
And graciously you stayed.

Sylvia Lynd

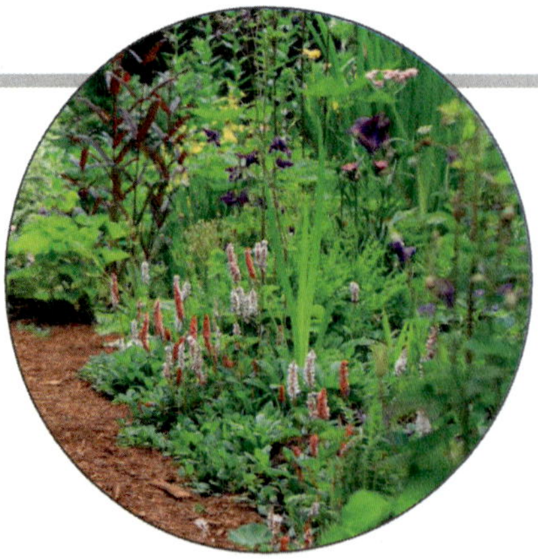

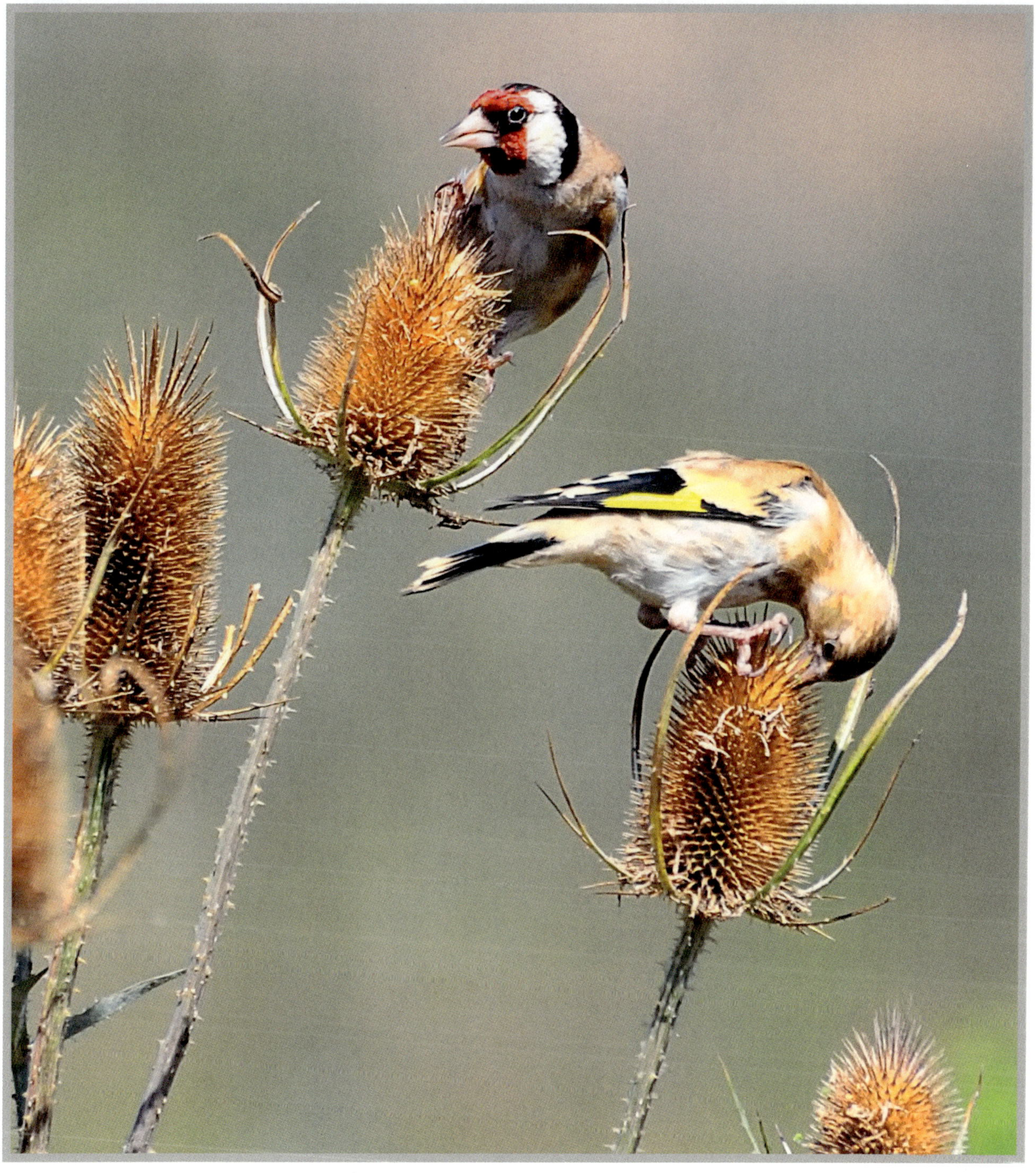

Dusk in June

Evening, and all the birds
In a chorus of shimmering sound
Are easing their hearts of joy
For miles around.

The air is blue and sweet,
The few first stars are white,—
Oh let me like the birds
Sing before night.

Sara Teasdale

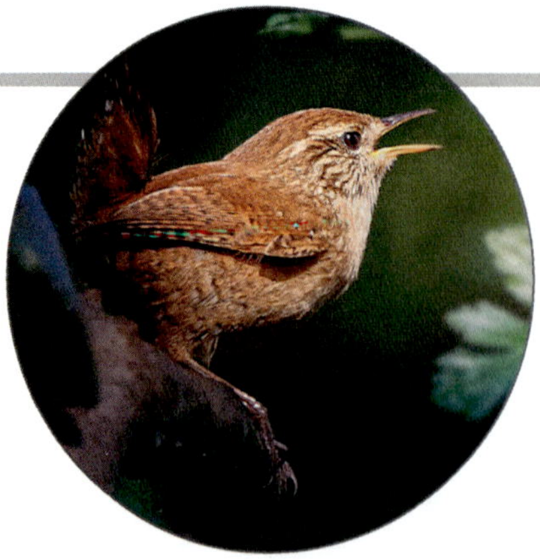

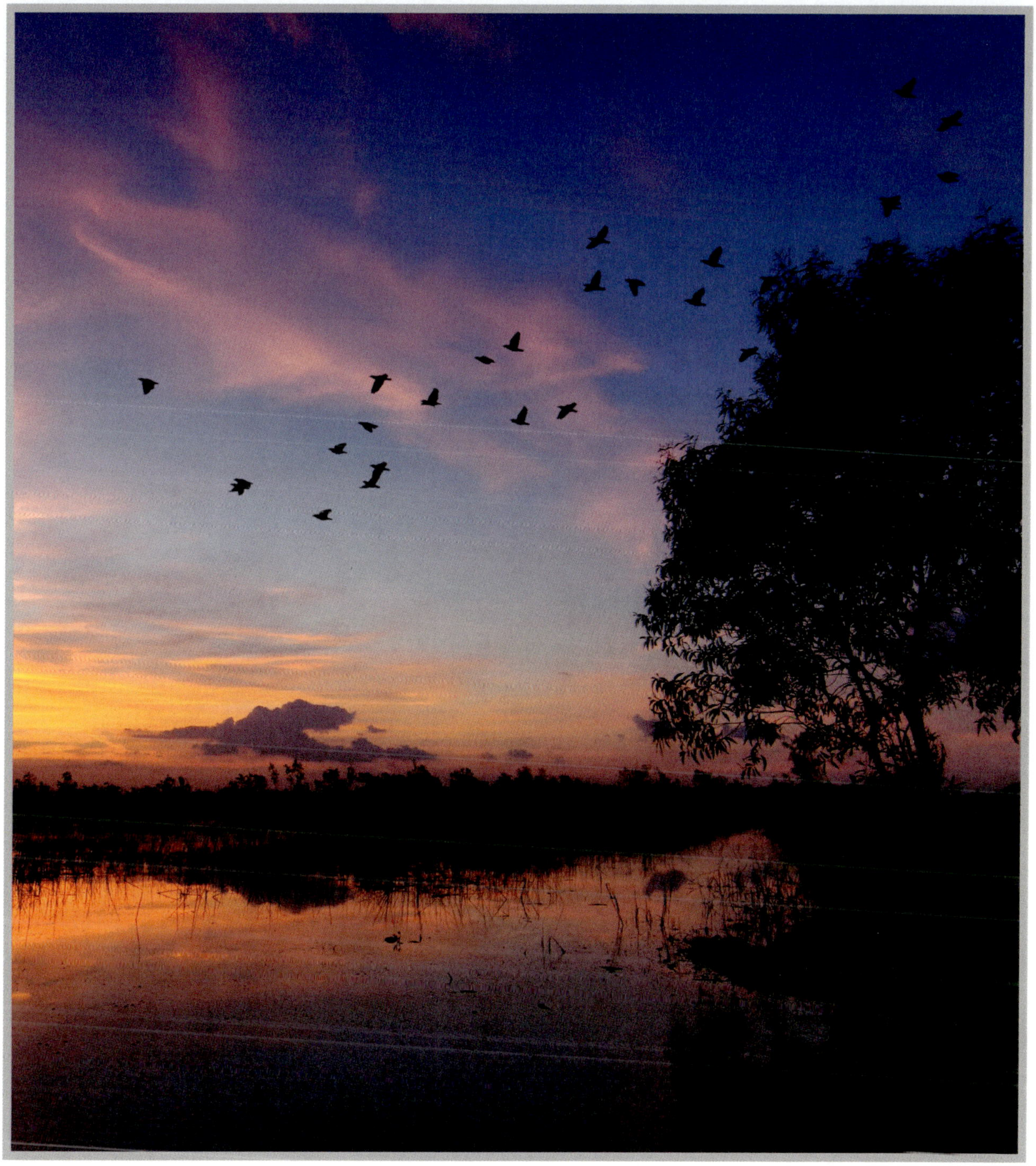

The Carrier Dove

If you have a carrier-dove
  That can fly over land and sea;
And a message for your Love,
  "Lady, I love but thee!"

And this dove will never stir
  But straight from her to you,
And straight from you to her,
  As you know and she knows too.

James Thomson

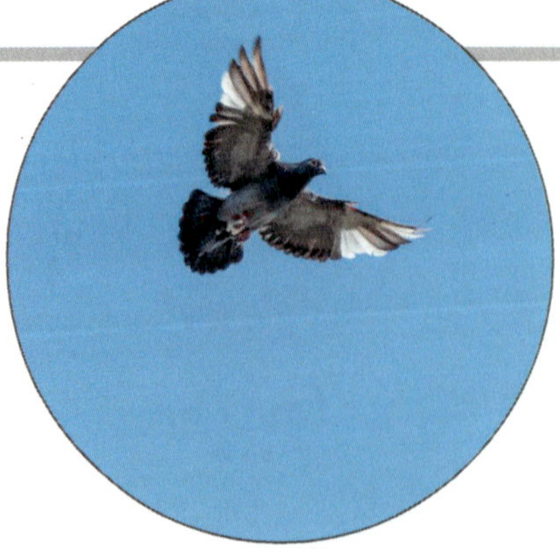

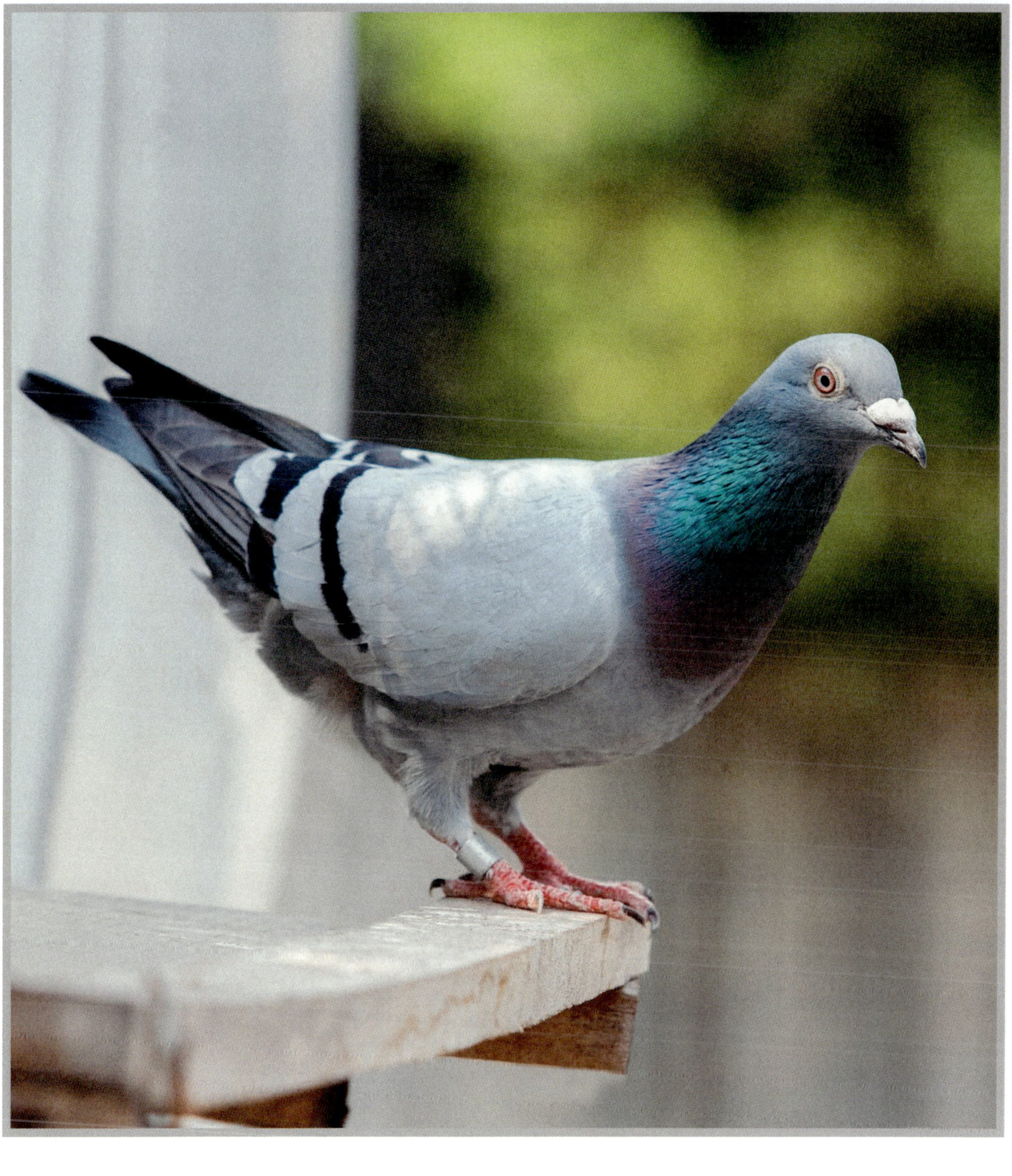

The Language of Birds

Do you ask what the birds say?
    The Sparrow, the Dove,
The Linnet and Thrush say, “I love and I love!”
In the winter they’re silent—
    the wind is so strong;
What it says, I don’t know, but it sings a loud song.
But green leaves, and blossoms,
    and sunny warm weather,
And singing, and loving—all come back together.

Samuel Taylor Coleridge

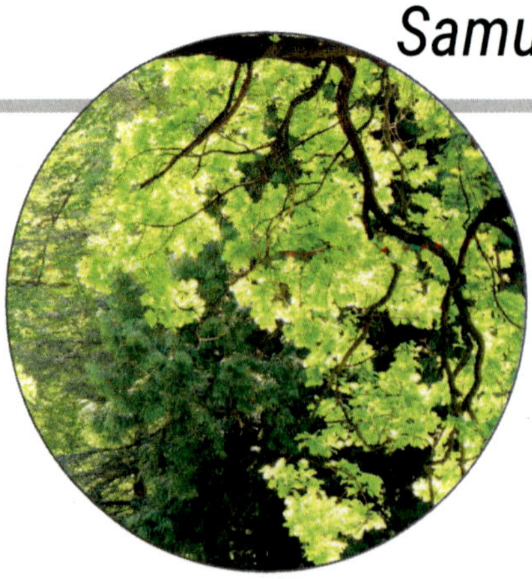

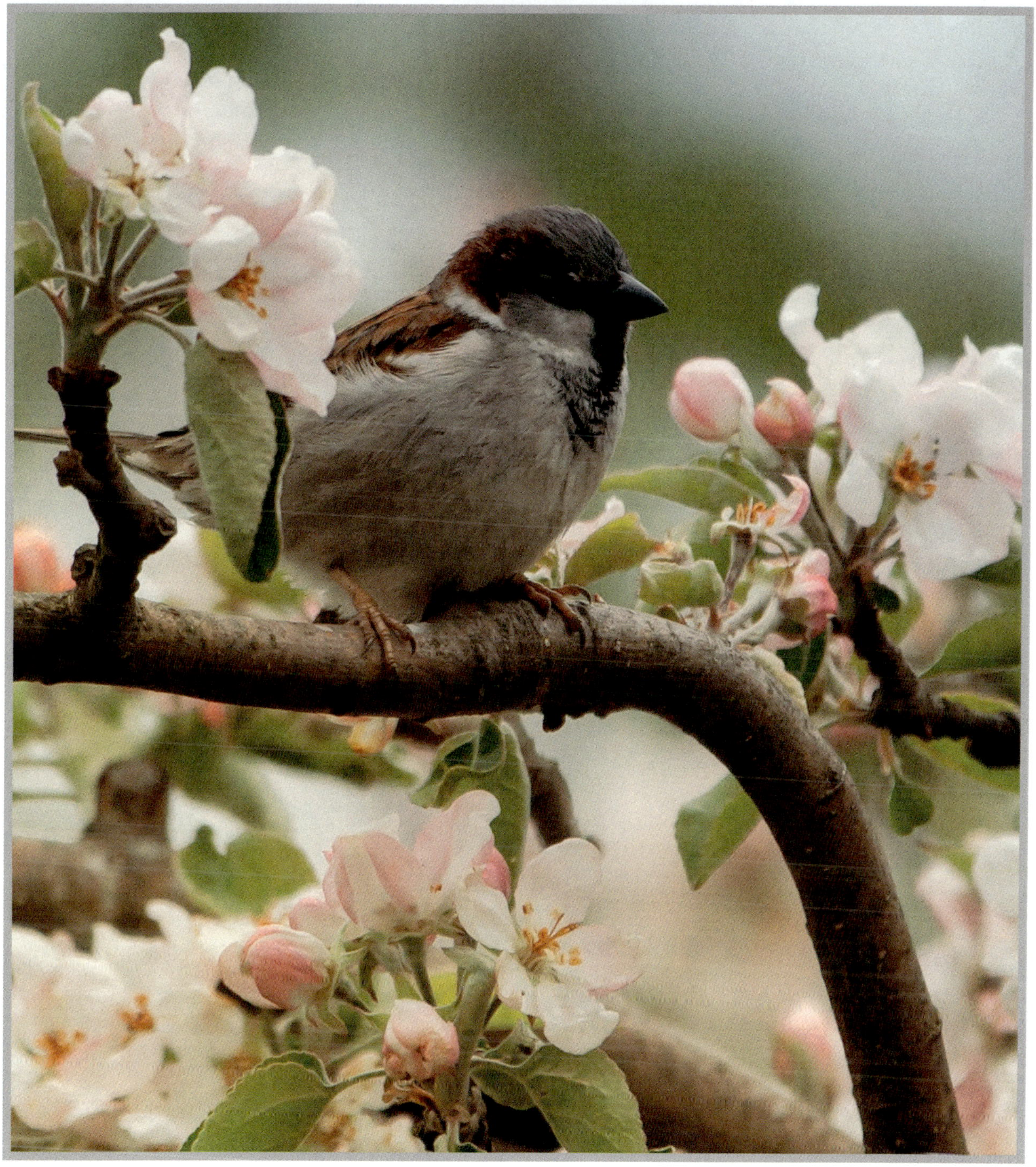

The Mockingbird

In mirth he mocks the other birds at noon,
Catching the lilt of every easy tune;
But when the day departs he sings of love,—
His own wild song
beneath the listening moon.

Henry Van Dyke

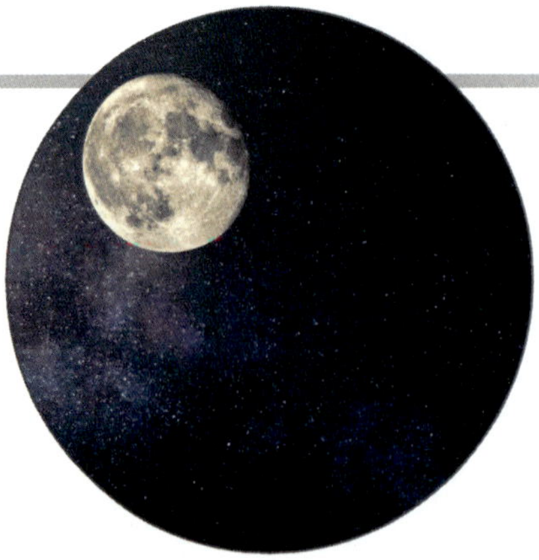

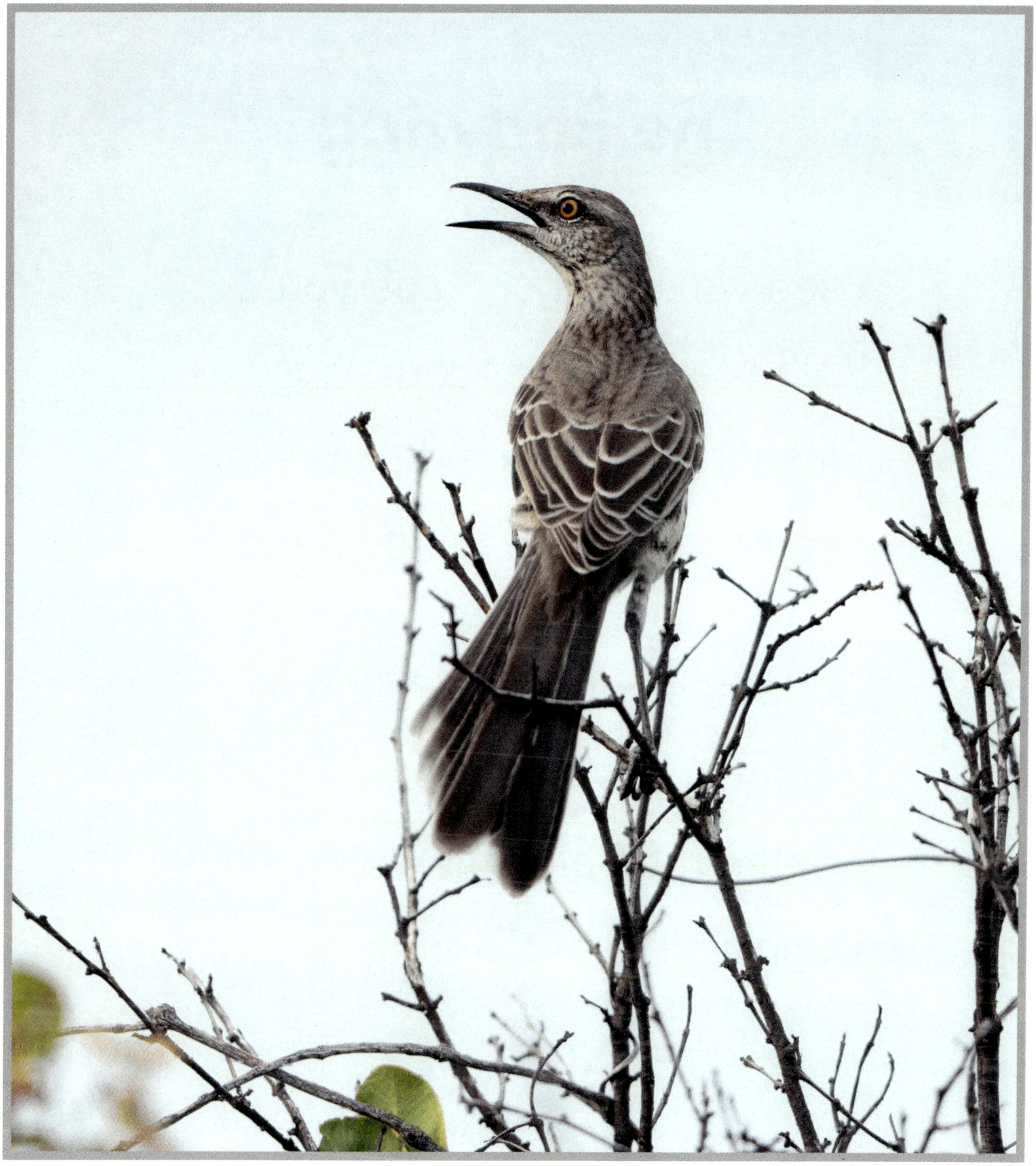

The Redwing

I see you, Brother, I see you,
With scarlet under your wing,
Flash through the ruddy maples,
Leading the pageant of spring.

Earth has put off her raiment
Wintry and worn and old,
For the robe of a fair young sibyl,
Dancing in green and gold.

Bliss Carman

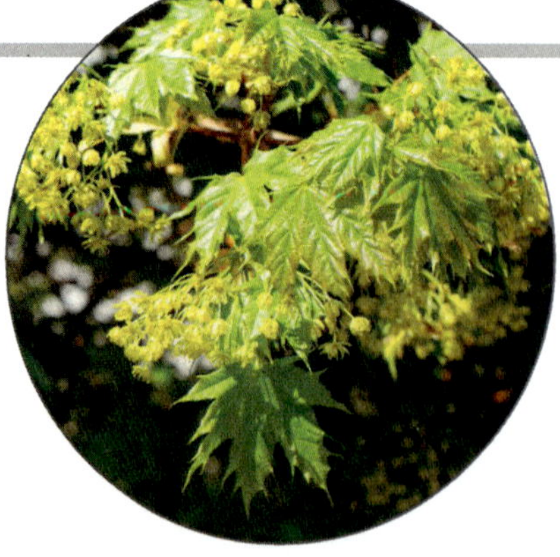

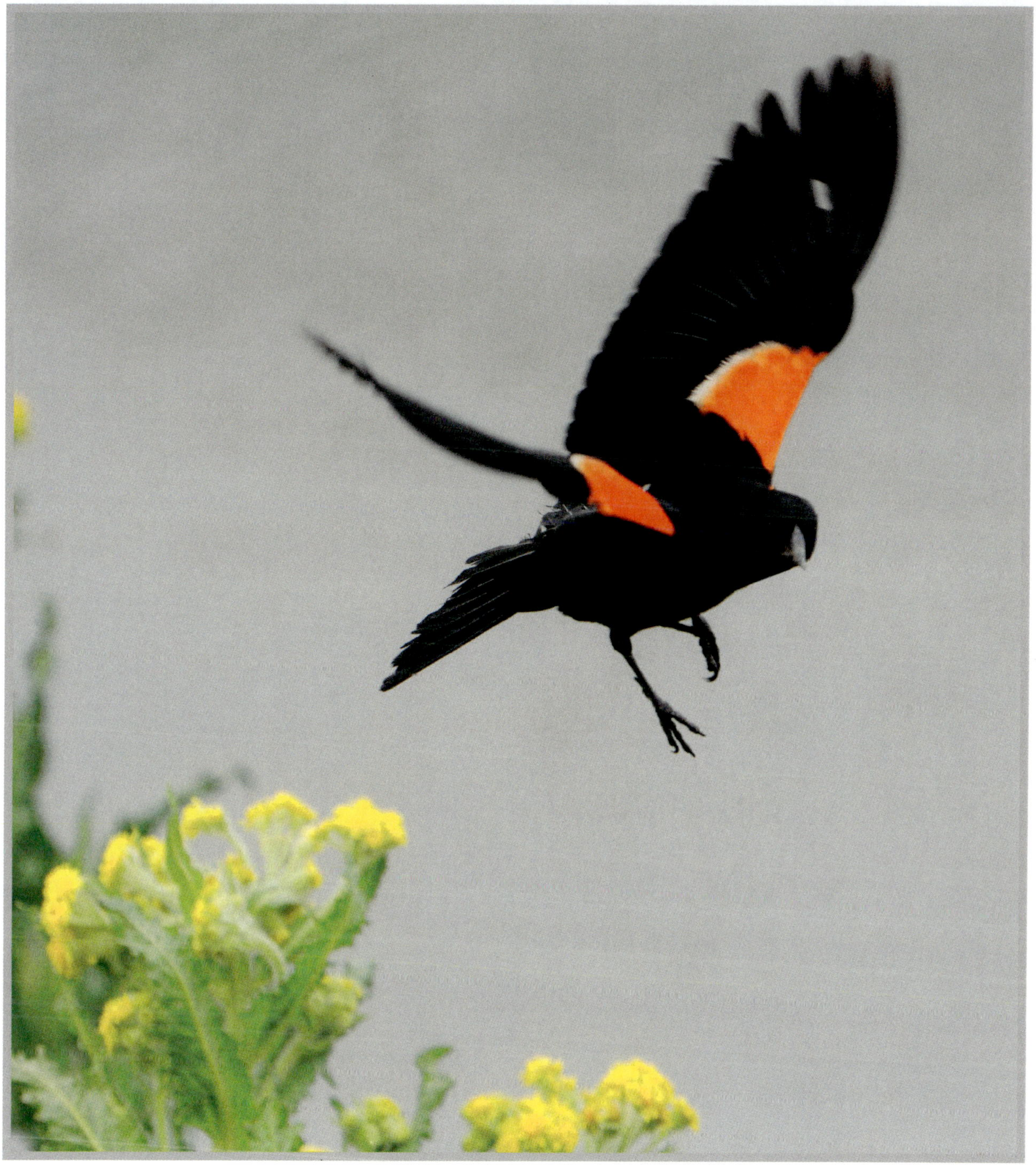

Sweet Birds, I come

The bird that now
On bush and tree,
Near leaves so green
Looks down to see
Flowers looking up—
He either sings
In ecstasy
Or claps his wings.

W. H. Davies

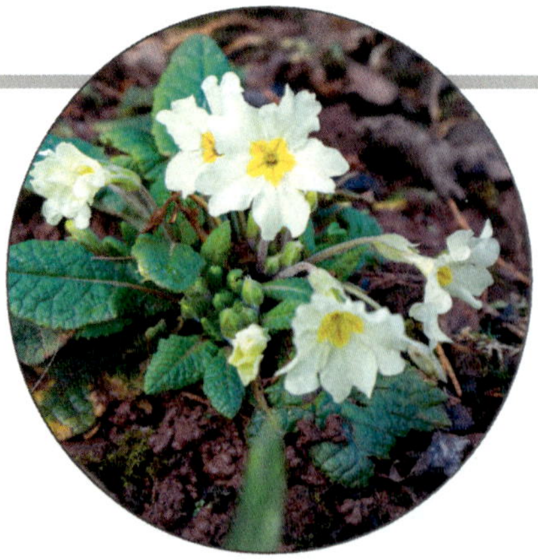

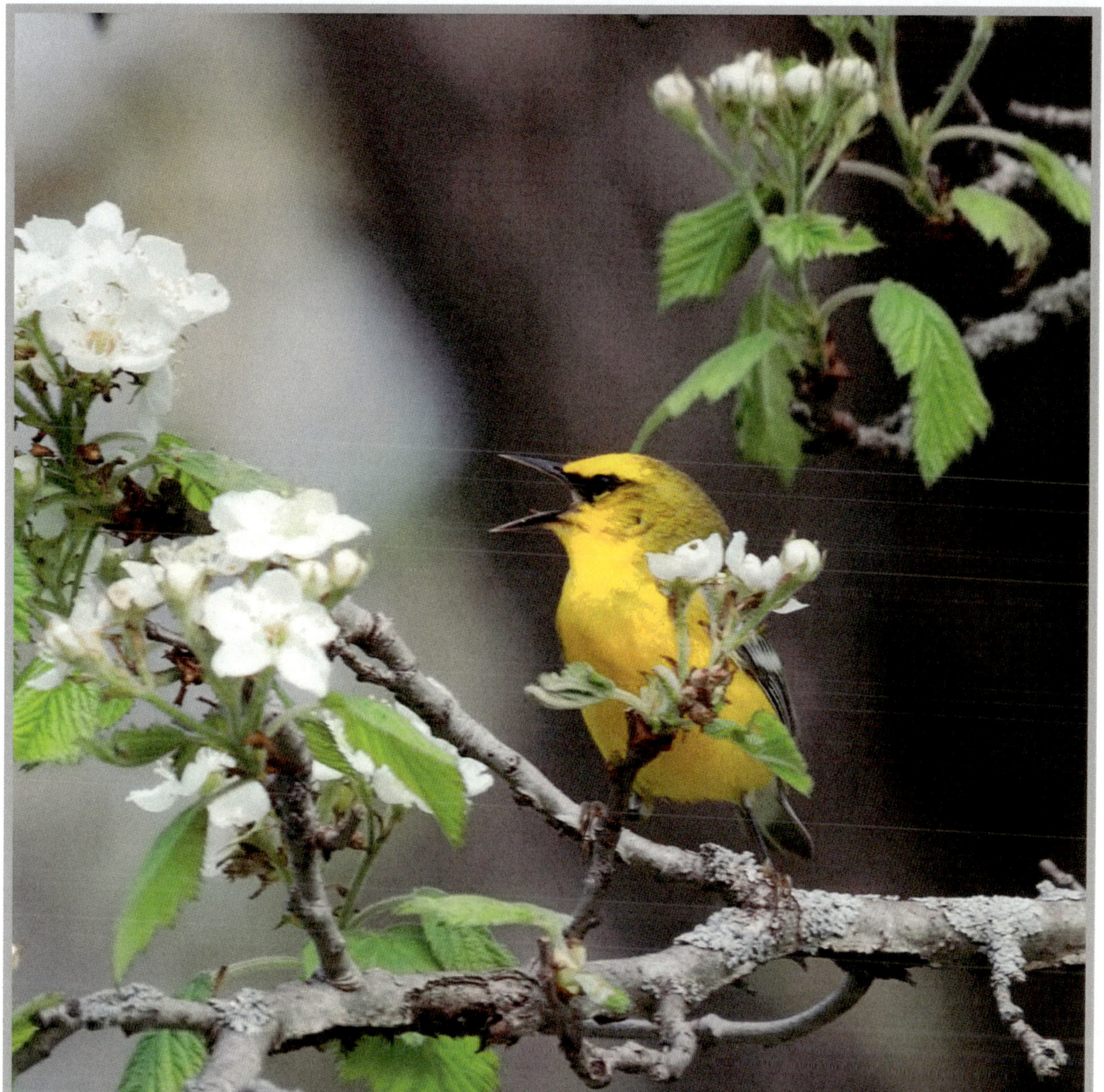

Thank you for reading!
You might also enjoy:

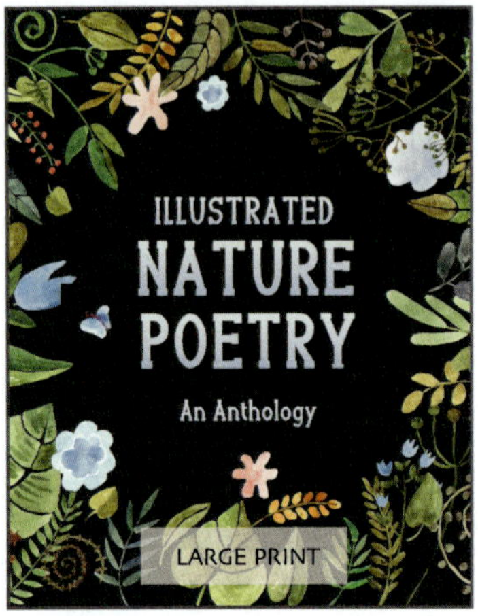

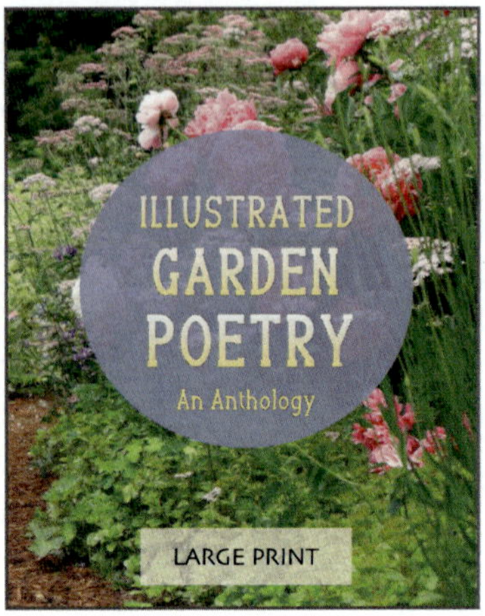

Huge thanks to Alison Egan (professional advice), Emma Laybourn, Jennifer J. Barwick (editing).

All these much-loved poems are in the Public Domain,
Photos from Deposit Photos:
majorosl66, Sandermeertinsphotography, dvoevnore, jiri_hrebicek, Elenatres, coboflupi, silver john, MarkCauntPhotography, Morrbyte, KeithPritchard, Xalanx, mikelane45,vencav, Hanjo Hellman, 205photog, khudoliy, travelwitness, callidusvisio, Perreten, Villam Mucha,BerndBrueggemann, scooperdigital, sport active, SarahLouPhotography, AOosthuizen, KeithPritchard, hannamariah, StockPhotoAstur, wirestock_creators, nirutdps, fotocorn, Khunaspix, Azjoma, Lincikas, Baranov_Evgenii, feather0510, Wirestock, pictureguy, Max_555, mtruchon

Made in the USA
Coppell, TX
05 November 2026

11302981R00026